# Acknowledgements

*I want to start by thanking my wonderful daughter, Tiana. Being your mom is the hardest and best thing in life. You gave me purpose when I was lost and I am truly grateful. You are the one person that has shaped who I am and you are my destiny. For better or for worse, you're my one true commitment that only you can bring into my life.*

*I want to thank my grandfather for setting the example of the person I want to be and dreamed of wanting to become. Him and my grandmother taught me how to nurture and heal. He gave me the skills that I would use for the rest of my life. I always have a place to go back to and feel grounded when I think of them. He is my inspiration for CoZi Skincare.*

*Writing this book has been on my mind for years. None of this would have been possible without my love, Davy. He has been so supportive and loving. He stood by me during every struggle and all my successes. This is a true relationship and one I will cherish forever.*

*Writing a book about the story of your life's work is a surreal process. I'm forever indebted to Chanet Smith for her editorial help, keen insight, and ongoing support in bringing my stories to life. Without her, this book would not have happened. I seek perfection, so creating a book was very challenging for me to write it in the right way. Thank you for resonating with me and understanding me. You've transformed my words into the way I've envisioned them. I am so grateful for our natural connection and trust in each other.*

*I want to thank EVERYONE who has impacted my life, advised me, motivated me, and taught me. I've heard all your kind words and they will stay with me forever. To my beautiful clients, thank you for trusting in me. Thank you for your loyalty. And thank you you for letting me be a small part of your life journey.*

*I want to grasp this opportunity for me to share my story. It's such a gift to have something you want to share with the world. I want to motivate women around the world to feel like they CAN and they WILL do whatever they set their minds on.*

**Self love: it's never too late to learn**

# Table of Contents

# Introduction

I grew up in a rice farm in rural Taiwan with my siblings, parents, and grandparents. My grandfather, whom I draw my inspiration from, was the rice farmer growing all the different vegetables and fruits of the seasons. We ate everything from farm to table and completely organic. After having my first child at a young age, I found comfort in being an aesthetician, a job I could learn at 17. My first clientele were my friend's moms and teens from my neighborhood and word of mouth. I dealt with a lot of severe acne and all I wanted to do was heal them. I also did a lot of bridal makeup, taking care of brides to-be all the way from a year prior to their wedding until their wedding day. I have a real soft spot for brides!

My first official job was creating facial testing protocol for a skincare manufacturing company. I delved into this experience of learning about ingredients, products, and what works well for the skin. It absolutely fascinated me to learn this process of skincare and ingredients! At 18, I opened my first spa under a company franchise inside my house. My daughter was 2 years old at this time, and I wanted to be closer and more available to her. The founder of the franchise was a chemist and he has a skincare manufacturer and a team of plastic surgeons that were focused as a medical spa. This company also had a branch for detox spa programs that was known for their "before" and "afters." People would check-in for their ten days to drink juice, take supplements, exercise classes. They had a class for everything, like mental health to yoga to fitness. I learned so much about internal health and detoxing under this company.

Afterwards, I worked closely with a company in Taiwan that imported Swiss skincare products and essential oils. They provided products to many of the spas in Taipei at the time. I was asked to be the team member to go to Switzerland and help clients with their treatment of sheep placenta injections which delays aging. It is a 7-10 day process that requires multiple injections, and the clients needed someone there with them through their treatment. My English was not good enough to work on an international scale, so I had to turn down this opportunity. It inspired me to learn English seriously, and my interest in America sparked. It was my goal to strengthen my skills and language to work in the international market. So off I went to America at 23 with one suitcase, $20,000, no English, and my ambition. And here I am, 22 years later, thriving in San Francisco.

I went back to aesthetician school in 2005 for the second time to strengthen my
technique and learn more in my field of expertise. I was hired as a lead aesthetician at St Regis Hotel Remede spa and trainer for the newcomers. It was such an amazing experience and I felt my confidence in my career was really taking off! After many years of working there, I felt it was time to open my own spa, where I could practice and work in my comfort zone and clientele. Running my own spa inspired me to create my own product line, one that incorporated my values, knowledge, and years of research. Now, after thirty years in the spa  industry, I carry my own line, CoZi Skincare, and run CoCo Spa by CoZi Skincare.

I believe skincare is definitely under healthcare. To me, having a trustworthy aesthetician is like having your dentist. It's something we all have and learn to manage whether it be acne, aging, dry skin, brown spots, etc. Just like you go to your dentist for check-ups and teeth cleaning, you should go to an aesthetician for the same reasons. In a professional treatment, I am able to address issues and use professional grade products and active ingredients that you can't use at home. And on top of that, I can analyze your skin and create a regimen for you at home that will be most effective rather than self-diagnosing and self-prescribing products. When you're shopping for skincare, most people stop for the pretty packaging and good marketing. This drives me crazy! These companies don't do a lot of "hands on" to figure out what the skin needs. They're based on research analytics of what people buy the most. They might have a great facility or chemist, but it's very hard to know what a skin needs unless you touch them and analyze the skin condition. We are all guilty of buying the product with the pretty bow rather than the product with the right ingredients.

In all, every person's skin is different, every person has different reactions, every person ages differently, and every person has different goals they want to reach for their skin. My everyday job is to touch people's faces, analyze them, and help them solve their skin concerns. How I treat their skin depends on their age, their genetics, their skin tone, their lifestyle, their ethnicity. I'm truly proud to be a skincare expert because I just learn so much on how things really affect the skin and I get to see these results and transformations time and time again.

Through all my years of experience, my strongpoints in the treatment room are really in pigmentation, acne, and extraction. I focus highly on preventative care for anti-aging and acne. My product line's strongpoints reflect my years of testing ingredients for what works best to solve the issues I see in the treatment room. I'll expand on my products more later in the book and I invite you to check my website coziskincare.com for more information on me, what I do, and my all -natural products.

# So...What is CoZi?

As an aesthetician, we must naturally be a nurturer. I truly care about my clients and their well-being. I listen to what they need from me professionally, but also create a safe place for them personally. What I have learned from them coming in for their treatments is that their head space and energy are just as important as the physical work that I do for them. I try to achieve all their goals, not just provide a service, and that is how CoZi Skincare was born. CoZi Skincare is vegan, paraben-free, and all-natural. I think the brand represents everything that I stand for: trust, comfort, cleanliness, and consistency. Our goal is to spread 'a little CoCo everywhere."

Working in the spa industry, I see a lot of massage therapists have skin disorders because they touch lotions with harsh chemicals all day long. I started to get very curious about "Why is their skin breaking out like that?" And it wasn't just once, it was a recurring issue for them. A lot of the older estheticians would get sick often and not know what was going on with them. No one was talking about safety in the spa industry for the spa therapists. Everyone working in the spa is surrounded by these luxurious products so no one was questioning the harmful effects they could be causing. It seemed to be just a way of life that went without question. When people would touch my hands, they say, "Oh my God, your hands are so soft., You're so lucky you get to touch the product all day long!" I started thinking, 'that's true. I touch products all day long with all those chemicals." I'm not just putting the products on my skin day and night, I'm working with it all day long. I got scared because I have always been very health conscious. Growing up, I watched my mom not take care of herself. She was always working in business, and due to that she passed away at 42. It made me realize how important it is to take care of your health.

My number one priority has always been about health. That's why I eat very healthy. That's why I exercise and cook primarily at home. That's why I try to do anything in my life around my health and wellness. And most importantly, that's why I started my own skincare line. It's so unhealthy to see so many product lines have all these harsh chemicals in them. I believe skincare on all levels can be nurtured through good eating habits and good products. I hold a very high standard to what I use and put into my body. It's all about the ingredients and the results.

I mostly gain my clientele from referrals. Being a boutique spa, I don't advertise, but work off of 'word-of-mouth.' I like growing my clientele organically because I want to attract like-minded people, wanting to care for their skin. It's nice to treat people that want to go beyond just a facial. The home part of this whole formula is so important and following a regimen. CoZi provides consumers with the right tools that they need at home, so they can be a part of the process of reaching their skin goals. And I'm happy to hear that my clients think this way too!

*"CoCo is magical. Previous to CoCo, I've been through 4+ aestheticians for facials in the last few years (and they all had 4 stars and up on yelp). It's usually a bad sign when you know more about skincare products than your aesthetician. It's especially bad when they push product that clearly don't work for your skin.*
*CoCo truly customizes facials and skincare regimens tailored to your skin. I've never seen anyone so meticulous, dedicated, detail-oriented, soothing and nurturing as this woman. She used to be on the product side before moving to aesthetic services, and she definitely knows her ingredients in skincare. She is also one of the best extractors I've seen. I have small pores, and I never scar even from some very tough extractions. In the last 3 times I've seen her, the few acne scars have all but vanished. My skin always glows after her visit.*
*She has her own skincare line as well. As a Korean beauty junkie who follows the latest skincare trends, her skincare line is a steal for the price and quality. If I didn't have all these other organic, vegan Korean skincare products in my cabinet, I would definitely use a few things from her line. She gave me a sample of the Vitamin A cleanser, and it definitely holds up to my cult faves from Korea." - Koh K.*

*"Wow Coco saved my skin!*

*I suffer from severe eczema on my face and Nothing I've tried in the past ,Reduced it so quickly .*
*It's been 1 week since I started on her fabulous Products , and my face looks the best it's have in months ..Her products are the real deal ..Happy Client" - Keithen B.*

*"I love Coco! I've been coming to Coco for a few years now and she really is the best! She's the only facialist I've been to where I don't break out after the fact. Also, her products are amazing. I've always had very dry skin and struggled to find products to keep it moist but her products do the trick!" - Alx N.*

<u>**Let's Talk Skin-Types**</u>

I first want to break down a few of the most common skin-types. It's important to know which type you are because the ingredients, regimens, and foods you're supposed to eat are all based on this! Understanding your skin-type is the first step to healthier skin.

☐ Aging

Aging skin is fine lines, wrinkles, sagging skin, and aging spots. It is basically when your skin loses its elasticity. As we get older, our skin naturally gets thinner. There are a lot of facts about genetics with aging skin. If your skin is more on the dry side it is going to age more and faster because your skin needs more nutrition than other skin-types. Some other factors that make you age faster are going under the sun, stress-levels (look at America's presidents before and after their term!), and if your diet doesn't have balanced nutrition. So unfortunately, skin tone is a big factor in aging. It's not always because you took better or worse care of your skin! Sun damage really affects lighter skin tone more, causing lighter tones to age faster. Many of my clients that have darker skin age better than lighter skin tones due to the melanin in their skin. When you go under a skin analysis machine, you can see deeper into your skin structure, pigmentation, brown spots, and the aging structure start to begin. Preventing aging is the key!

Aging skin is all about prevention. Use products that are antioxidant rich. The CoZi Anti-aging Serum has fibroblast growth factors. It is from amino-rich extract of hibiscus to help stimulate collagen production. It also has apple stem cell ingredients to promote the upper layer skin cells. Our CoZi Blueberry Cream has high antioxidants like blueberries, grape skins, and green tea extracts. A new trend right now is doing Gua Sha massage on your face to promote the circulation in your skin. It is a marketing scam! If you don't pull your skin in the proper direction or over-do it, you are damaging your face and pulling your skin in the wrong direction.

This will actually cause saggy skin rather than stimulate anti-aging benefits. Moral is: learn how to do it CORRECTLY.

A client of mine is a very well-known ballet dancer in the principal of San Francisco Ballet. She is in my testimonials on my website. I love talking about her as an example of preventative aging because her skin just looks amazing. She has been coming to me for 13 years now consistently and she looks the same as when I met her in 2006. I try to educate my younger clients to start being proactive in their anti-aging now! It's as simple as not going out to drink a couple of nights a week or -- a month, you could have saved the money to do a facial. If you think about a $6 coffee a day...that's $180 a month! That money can easily go towards a facial or quality skincare products. It's all about what you prioritize in your health and your life.

*"As a dancer, sweat and make-up must be cleared regularly, and CoCo has been the only one I trust my face and skin to. I have not found anyone that has understood my needs, healed my damages and prepared my skin the way CoCo does. She has an unusual capacity to adapt to every person's skin needs and the confident feeling you get walking out of her spa is priceless." – Sofiane Sylve, Principal Dancer for San Francisco Ballet*

☐ Pigmentation

Pigmentation is the brown spots on your skin. Majority of them come from being under the sun because melanin is produced to protect your skin from UV rays. Pregnancy also causes brown spots, sometimes in the shape of a butterfly because of the hormone imbalance. These pregnancy marks usually go away after you give birth. A lot of my clients that take birth control will end up with brown spots on their face and darker pigmentation around their forehead, lips and under the eyes called melasma. That's due to the hormone imbalance. Asian skin tones are the most common to have pigmentation and are the toughest to treat.

In these cases, a lot of people like to use brightening agents like hydroquinone, which has high safety concerns. It is already banned in Japan, the EU, and Australia. I suggest using the more natural ingredients like arbutin, kojic acid, and lactic acid for whitening and exfoliating the skin. The CoZi Vitamin A Cleanser carries lactic acid, and in the treatment room, I use a glycolic peel that has both arbutin and kojic acid. These help with brightening the skin because cherry and plum pulp are natural brighteners. I promote these natural brighteners because the truth about pigmentation is they will never disappear 100%. So if you want to treat it as an ongoing process, use something safer for your skin. From a preventative perspective, I always suggest avoiding the sun, wearing hats, and wearing SPF. Another important note is when you exfoliate – don't over exfoliate. Twice a week with a light exfoliator is the general amount you should be exfoliating. Over-exfoliating would be when you do lasering and peels because they remove many upper layers of skin. Our skin is good to protect you from external factors, so don't just rip it off!

The bottom line is you can always treat pigmentation to lighten up, but it will be more effective to think about pigmentation from a preventative perspective. They will naturally lighten up if they are not always stressed under the sun!

☐ Acne

It is really important for people with acne-prone skin type to have education from professionals for their skin to be healthier. When you are struggling with your skin, do not self-diagnose, go to dermatologists and aestheticians for professional help. The short-term solution to acne is antibiotics or accutane, but there are risks involved with this route. My focus is highly on preventive and proactive skincare. Most of my clients are acne clients because they need facials the most, and they learn from a younger age how to take care of their skin, from teenagers to adults of any age. Acne affects your self confidence and how you view yourself. A lot of women use birth control to control their acne and when they come off the pill, their acne starts appearing again. Menopause, stress, genetics, and diet are all factors of acne as well. I really focus on acne clients because I know how important it is to treat them, support them, and be there for them. It is a long process. It takes time and patience. My job is to change the blueprint of their skin, but they need to reconstruct the habits in their lives.

Acne can be broken down into levels 1-5. Acne 1-2 consists of blackheads, whiteheads and clogged pores. Acne 3-4 is more like inflamed pustules (common acne) and papules. Level 5 is cystic acne and nodules. Oily skin is not necessarily acne skin, it is just bigger pore sizes. Your overactive sebaceous glands don't have to cause acne if you keep good hygiene. (A plus: you generally age better when you have oily skin!) Acne mechanica is caused by friction, sweat, and heat. Wearing helmets, wearing backpacks, working out, and not washing your skin causes this type of acne. It is most common on your back, shoulder, and forehead. Throughout the day, oil and debris gets clogged into your pores, causing breakouts. The easiest way to cure this type of acne is simply just washing your skin after sweating or creating friction in that area. Try to steer clear of wearing heavy make-up or any at all, especially when working out!

I want to educate the younger generations because as an adult, we already build our routines and habits and it becomes harder to manage. If you have healthier skin younger, you feel better with your self-confidence and wear less make-up, etc. When you have acne, you don't have a privilege to just do whatever everyone else is doing. It affects your confidence when you don't have good skin. It affects you as a young person growing up. Knowing how to treat it earlier on can prevent a lot of that. It's a lot about health, not so much beauty. When you're young, you don't take the time to think about your skin and pores in those moments until acne starts showing up. Therefore, when you're young, it's really important to learn simple habits and have the right products. It doesn't have to be expensive or complicated. Learn to wash your face day and night, use a toner because it helps balance the pH. Even water has higher alkaline levels than your pH levels.

Inflammation can be caused by certain foods such as dairy, gluten, and sugar. When I treat acne clients, I focus highly on changing their diet. I don't just say, "come get a facial and use this product." For the younger generation, I like to look at their stress levels, their hormones, and recommend they check with a dermatologist or doctor. It's extremely important to get to the root of the problem. For people with the financial means, I suggest they go to an esthetician regularly for their skin concerns. I like to create a program for them because it isn't a 'one-time facial and they're cured'. It will be a long-term commitment. My program makes sure they only use the products I suggest and make sure they are committed to the lifestyle changes required by the program, to watch their stress levels, and change their diet. They need to be on top of their at-home regimen as well. I even require them to work out with no make-up and wash their face directly after.

Acne doesn't just appear on the face, but the neck, chest, decollate area, back, etc and can be so painful when it is inflamed. In some cases, clients need to come in every week or two to do extraction on their pores. Of course this helps the skin short-term, but it doesn't solve the issue. Be on top of it. I try to change the blueprint of my client's skin so there is a more successful chance of treating it. It is so important to NOT PICK. Picking can be a habit when you are stressed or thinking. The reason why you pick is because it's THERE and it's congested. If there is no acne, then you don't have to pick it. My goal is to have them come in for extraction before they reach the point of picking. I help my clients to do a 21 day challenge where I hold them accountable to not picking. They send me a text and a picture of their face to let me know they're not picking. Just like quitting smoking. Something that you can do for 21 days has a better chance of breaking that habit. I always say to drink herbal teas like chamomile to calm and relax yourself rather than going at your face.

With acne, it is super important in using the right product for your acne condition. That is really EVERYTHING when curing it! Salicylic Acid, Sulfur, and Benzoyl Peroxide, Tea Tree Oil, Arnica are great ingredients to look for in your acne products. CoZi blemish control cleanser carries salicylic acid, pumpkin extract, clove oil, and it emulsifies with the oil and debris on your face throughout the day and removes very gently without stripping the healthy oil from your skin. So it's really good for cleaning your skin gently, but effectively. It also has AHA, which gently exfoliates your skin daily. The CoZi Anti-Blemish mask carries Sulfur, and CoZi Anti-Blemish moisturizer has both Tea Tree Oil and Arnica. Using these products together in your regimen will drastically help your acne. Always include a good toner in your regimen that DOESN'T have alcohol in it!

*"I've been coming to CoCo for a little over a year now. I'm so happy that I have been coming. All my life I have had problematic skin. I've been getting regular facials since I was 15. Since I have been coming here, I have seen so much more improvement. My skin has gotten a lot better in terms of less breakouts and better skin texture. Now I am excited that I can wear NO makeup on weekends and feel happy, confident and beautiful. I am so excited. I really really really love CoCo and I am so happy I found her! It is so hard to find a good esthetician, so when you find one, you need to hold on to them and never leave them! I am even scared to leave San Francisco because I don't know what is going to happen when I leave!" - Khadine Singh, young professional in San Francisco*

☐  Dry

The biggest complaint with dry skin is it is ALWAYS dry. It feels hopeless no matter how many products you try, how much moisturizer you put on, and how much water you drink. Dry skin is mostly genetic and caused by health issues like hypothyroidism. Dry skin can be associated with aging due to the unwelcome wrinkles that start coming in. A common misconception of dry skin is pounding on heavy moisturizers or using many different hydrating products.

To start, only wash your face at night. It is important to not overstrip your natural oils. Use lukewarm water, not hot, not cold. With dry skin, the key is layering hydrating products to get a moisturized effect. Using a heavy moisturizer will just build up on top of your skin, not able to penetrate into your pores. Use a product with Hyaluronic acid (natural occurring molecule in our skin) and QUALITY hydrating serums. Hyaluronic is really the key ingredient because the molecule holds 1,000 times its weight in water and is retained in our skin. It's an amazing hydrating ingredient. And on top of that, we naturally have hyaluronic acid in our body, but as we age it gets lower and lower. Exfoliating is best for dry skin because it helps your skin absorb serums and products better. Always use toner right after washing your face because it helps balance your PH. If you have cracking skin, especially on the hands, my favorite product to use is simply Neosporin. A very good body hydrator is organic coconut oil on your hair and body, but not on the face! You don't need to buy special 'body-type' coconut oils, just pure organic coconut oil.

I recommend the CoZi Enzyme Peel because it has bananas, pineapple, and papaya enzymes to dissolve dead skin, but is NOT abrasive. I call this product our little monster because it eats the dead skin off of you! My number one best-seller is the CoZi Collagen Mask because it works on dry skin and aging skin like no other product does. Many of my clients use it as an overnight mask to maximize penetration. It has plant-based collagen, Jojoba, sunflower seed oil, and Vitamin E and C.

*Remember the key to curing dry skin is layering hydrating products and using a quality serum! Don't fall for a thick moisturizer!


☐   Sensitive
Majority of people have sensitive skin. It's just a matter where they are on a scale of 1-10. Sometimes it can be caused by a chronic health issue, which causes inflammation and sensitivity. Your skin will become more sensitive if you are: over-exfoliating,

over-treating, washing your face too much, laser treatments, harsh chemical products, over-exposing to the sun, seasonal change, or going through menopause. When you have acne and treat it with harsh chemicals, your skin will become more sensitive as well. You HAVE to be extra nurturing with sensitive skin. It isn't just a problem, there is a reason your skin is sensitive. Be compassionate to your sensitive skin.

The most common type of clients I get with sensitive skin are rosacea clients. Then after that are clients with dermatitis and eczema. To treat this skin-type, take lukewarm showers because heat activates sensitivity. Use gentle body washes and face washes, even hair products!  This affects your skin everywhere. I would recommend only washing your face at night rather than in the morning and night. Only use showergel once a day if you shower more than once a day. Basically, DON'T over-use products because that is what is irritating your skin. Gentle, fragrance-free, simple ingredient products are key with sensitive skin. Sensitive skin is highly reactive to many ingredients, especially active ingredients. The best ingredients for sensitive skin are chamomile extract, aloe vera, and Calendula extract.

☐  Rosacea

Rosacea is a genetic disease that many people use medication to regulate, as it is a lifetime issue. It doesn't just go away. Incorporating it into your lifestyle will help you manage it much better. Avoiding very hot weather, staying cool, taking lukewarm showers will help on the surface of your skin. Internally, focus on avoiding spicy foods and alcohol, as these are triggers for your condition. Incorporate anti-inflammatories into your diet that will help keep your condition under control.

In the treatment room, I use an LED light to not over stimulate blood flow. The LED light is great for rosacea because it helps penetrate the product deeper down, without irritating the skin on top, opposed to massaging the skin. I try not to massage too much because it will create redness and irritation along the surface. What I try to tell people with rosacea is: Don't try to fix it, try to live with it.

<u>**Finding Your Regimen**</u>

For a daily routine, I suggest a  cleanser, toner, serum, eye cream, and moisturizer. For weekly, it would be an exfoliator and a mask. It depends on your skin type that you can define which product to use, how much of it, and whether to add/subtract from that routine. I always analyze my client's at-home skin regimen to see what is working and what isn't. From there, we can change the products or the usage to better fit what their skin is wanting. Everyone has 'their product' they love for over ten years and they don't want to change it. That's totally fine, but defining skin and what it needs is my expertise. As an esthetician, I can professionally give advice, suggestions, and knowledge to simply organize your skin regimen better at home. There are so many factors to a product working FOR YOU. Climate, travel, stress, age, diet...these are all factors that change regularly.

I have a client with acne in the T-zone area that was very oily and very dry at the same time. When she used acne products, her skin would get dryer. When she used oil products, her skin would break out more. I recommended her to not use oil or heavy moisturizer when her skin feels dry, but a toner and hydrating serum instead. Serum penetrates the skin better than a moisturizer. These are small changes in your at-home regimen that make a huge difference in your daily life.

My philosophy with skincare is all about preventive AND proactive. It is true, you can never be too late, but what if you can slow down your aging for ten years, why not? Right? I recommend using SPF every day! When you apply it once, it only lasts for an hour or two, so keep re-applying! If you know you're going to be out in the sun all day, instead of worrying about constantly re-applying, just wear a hat! Don't have your face directly in the sun. For you sunlovers, direct sunlight causes wrinkles and pigmentation (brown spots) to come much faster.  The key here is to age gracefully through healthier skin.

☐   Overwhelmed With the Skincare Market

When you are shopping for your products, there are three keys to look for with anything you want to buy. Make sure it is gentle on the skin. Make sure it is fragrance-free. Make sure the ingredient list is simple. When you have scented products, check if it is artificial or real. Chemical scents are not good for your skin, especially when you are fighting acne, dry skin, and sensitive skin. I suggest gentle products because you are using it on your face every day. If you are using a harsh scrub or an alcohol product, every single day it is rubbing onto your skin and stripping away its barrier function. I say 'simple ingredients' again because of chemicals.

Many of us get so overwhelmed with skincare because it is always in your face all day every day! On your phone, your computer, at the store, marketing pops up all day long. People just believe it so easily because it really is good marketing. BUT, good marketing does not mean a good product, and a good product doesn't always mean that it will be right for you. For example, the subscription box. It works well with material things like clothes, shoes, but when it comes to skincare, I highly highly recommend not to do the subscription box because every month they give you different products. If it was a subscription box for the same products, or even changing them seasonally would make sense, but don't change your products for your skin every month.

We have a natural skin barrier function. Naturally our bodies have a self-protecting mechanism. Our bodies know how to protect us from a harmful environment. That's why brown spots come up- to protect our skin from sun damage and UV rays. When you change your products every month, your skin is always in a state of shock, trying to figure out how it wants to react with the new products. To me, it's important to be more mindful about the ingredients and the amount of products we use on our faces. The different skin-types require different ingredient needs, like oily skin, T-zone oily, active oil glands, combination skin, dry skin, or sensitive skin. Majority of people have sensitive skin, but the range 1-10 will be different per person. So it is important that the products are catering to your skin-type.

It is really good knowledge to know your skin-type rather than just following trends and marketing. Skincare should not be all about marketing. All these big companies are trying to sell you something and be a part of a trend. Don't just keep going in that pattern. Just because it works for some people doesn't mean it will work for you too. That's what I do in the spa, I give education one at a time. But I want to do this book so I can give knowledge to more than one person at a time. When people come to me and ask about a product they are using, I can't just say "this product is better for you!" because I am very analytical and particular when it comes to products. That's why I created my own line! I have to put it on my skin, my clients skin, so I never suggest a product unless I have tried it before on my own skin. I can't just read ingredients and say, "oh this is good or use this product." I take pride in what I do every day. I check in with myself, is this helping others? Does this resonate with me? If I don't take pride in what I do every day then it can't be good for anyone, especially myself. Good things come from taking the time and doing it right.

It's all about who you trust and who you go to. A lot of beauty stores are an overwhelming corporate based market. They don't always know your best interests, but what sells the best. All I can say is research, research, research. We have unlimited tools at our fingertips these days to get as much knowledge about a product as we want! Use that to your advantage.

☐ Regimens
I have a client and she is really good at taking care of her skin, always getting new facials with all kinds of products. Yet, she comes to me every two weeks or month because she always has clogged pores and blackheads. I've been treating her for months and cleaning it all out, but then she comes back to me and is completely clogged again. I told her not to do these Korean 9-

step/12-step regimens because there are too many steps every day for her skin. It stresses the skin and barrier function. So I asked her to do me a favor to try and break her habit of always trying new products. Just use three products a day for a month, a cleanser, toner, and moisturizer. She said to me, "Can I do three different products for day and night?!". She loves her skincare products and has so many. But I told her she needs to try just three of the same products regularly for a month. She tried it and came back to me with no clogging! She was so happy that it worked.

The moral of that story is LESS is MORE! Your at-home DAILY regimen should be according to your skin-type and condition. When you're older, you might need more products to prevent aging. When you're younger, your skin does not need as much product. Daily routine is the most important thing you can do for your skin. This is where you have control. Don't waste your time with products that don't suit you. When you have a good regimen, you can even do your facial at home. It's just like eating food. To be better, you eat healthy and take supplements. Same thing for your skincare routine, have beneficial products that you use day and night for healthier skin.

# <u>Breaking Down Products</u>

Skincare regimen is like eating a balanced diet. You need a well thought-out process of what goes on your skin. Every product you include works for your skin in a different way. When investing in products, don't just read ingredients, but consider the history of the company and manufacturing. Is it ethical? Is it cruelty-free from animals? Was it tested for stability? Does it guarantee consistency and quality? If a product works well for your friend does not necessarily mean it will work well for you too. For younger people, they have a simpler routine, and when you are older, there are more steps to take. If you're acne prone, you need to have minimum products. I will explain each product in the order of which it should be used in. Every product serves a purpose in the order that you use it in. You don't want to moisturize your face without cleansing your skin first. What I recommend daily: a makeup remover, cleanser, toner, eye cream, moisturizer, and SPF. Weekly, exfoliation and a mask. Yes, you need eye cream even when you are young. To slow down aging, it's all about prevention. For some women, you need to put makeup on daily. If you don't have a good skin foundation to begin with, no amount of makeup is going to help you feel your best. With my clients, when they start feeling confident about their skin, they stop wearing all their face makeup because they are glowing without it.

My tips for DIY, they aren't always a good idea. Skin is very complex. It's easy to get a reaction out of any ingredient, even when it's natural. By all means, if you have a home remedy that works for you, then that's great! But for the majority of us, I would be cautious with what you read and see online to make home remedy skincare.

When picking your products, make sure to read the ingredients, and watch for 'active ingredients.' For example, glycolic acid, salicylic acid, and retinols are strong ingredients and can cause burning skin. Each of these ingredients serve a different purpose at different stages in your life. If you need to use these products, you NEED to be educated on how to use your products properly. For example, in the beginning of using retinol, you should be using it every three days at night time for the first two weeks. Once your skin is used to it, then you can use it every other day. This is an ingredient that varies based on skin-type. Overall, try to find a line that has a well thought out process for each product and how it complements each other and serves a purpose for your skin. With a line that has been tried and tested, you aren't overdoing the active ingredients in all the products in your regimen. What I suggest against is mixing and matching, like the subscription boxes that carry numerous brands. It's like, "Oh, that product is good, its great, I'm going to put all this stuff on my skin." But in reality, you don't know which one is really helping you, and before you know it, you have all new products to try. This can stress your skin out or have reactions from mixing certain ingredients.

The key steps of picking products:
1.  Go to a professional - they can analyze your skin and give you tips.
2.  Know your skin type - once you know this, you know what you'll need.
3.  Research products - if it fits not only your skin type, but also your ethical standard. Don't always believe social media and marketing of that product, do proper background research.
4.  Don't buy a full package - Products are expensive so try the samples. If the samples work out, then buy the product line. But set the intention of wanting to commit to one. I have seen the results of people that get in the habit of wanting to try samples of all different products regularly, and their skin is constantly irritated and breaking out.
5.  Stay consistent - Once you've found the golden product line, STICK WITH IT! Be cognisant that good products have a shelf life. Don't overstock at once, always make sure your products are coming in fresh.

*Side note: when you're travelling to different climates or there is a seasonal change, your skin is going to change with it. You might need a different product that will acclimate your skin to your environment.

## Makeup Remover

Some makeup has comedogenic ingredients which clogs pores and causes acne. When you're told to take your makeup off daily, it's due to these harsh ingredients of cosmetics. Makeup remover takes off the makeup, but also the oil and debris you've built up throughout the day. A common misconception is that remover is only for the eyes, but the most important part is your face, and removing cosmetics from your pores. A lot of people like to use oil or water-based makeup remover, which is fine, as long as you wash your face afterwards. Oil-based remover is good to break down mascara without damaging your eyelashes. CoZi Remover is water-based and can remove mascara that is not waterproof. You HAVE to use a cleanser after makeup remover because most makeup removers leave a residue of product ingredients on your face. People always ask me if they can use their cleanser as their makeup remover- just wash their face and skip this step. I would recommend makeup remover prior. Makeup remover is designed specifically to get off the harsh chemicals of their cosmetic products. For example, many of them have heavy metals, lead, and mineral oil as ingredients, which you don't want to leave on your skin. You want to remove that so your pores are clear for your cleanser.

## Cleanser

I get asked if cleanser and soap are the same thing or if one is better than the other. I would say it depends on the ingredients. Most soaps have less ingredients than cleansers, and that works for people that really need to control what ingredients they use. If you are looking for ingredients that are made for your skin-type, cleansers are the way to go. The CoZi Vitamin A Cleanser has pumpkin extracts and clove oil. It emulsifies the oil debris throughout the day without stripping the healthy oils. This type of emulsification prevents getting blackheads. I always tell my clients to wash their face when they get home from their day, not just before bed. No matter how tired you are, cleanse your skin at night if you aren't able to when you get home from work. For females, it's a double cleanse. You have to remove the makeup. Then you use the cleanser. They are separate products! Otherwise, I cannot tell you how many people still have their makeup, even if they say, "Oh, I washed my face, I showered. I have nothing on my face." Then you find makeup!

☐   Toner

Toner is commonly misunderstood of how it is used and why it is used. In Asia, we are trained to understand 'essence' which in the states we call toner. In the United States, people know toner as 'astringent', to remove extra oil in oily acne-prone skin. I always explain that toner is like drinking water for your face. It prevents environmental damage, and balances your skin to a healthy pH. People also think toner is to remove the residue. As a skincare professional, you should have a good cleanser to remove residue. Toner is like a bridge between your skin and your products. It enhances the products to absorb better. A good toner has NO alcohol. Many people think that alcohol is needed to fight acne, but it strips your skin's health and natural oils causing dehydration. Toner helps to balance the pH because water has a higher alkaline, especially for men that use a shaver. For example, shaving cream is a highly alkaline product. Normal water's pH is 6.5pH-8.5pH and healthy skin should be between 4.8pH-6pH. Toner helps bring you to that healthy medium around 5.5pH.

☐   Serums

Many people don't start to use serums until they are older. It's commonly mistaken to use a heavier moisturizer as an anti-aging preventative, but heavy moisturizers aren't good for every skin type. Serums have all the active ingredients concentrated into one product without petrolatum or mineral oil. A serum has smaller molecules to penetrate deeper into the skin with the most active ingredients (this is why it is more expensive!) A common ingredient in serums are stem cells. Stem cells are the newest and most popular active ingredient. They contain amino acids and peptides which are the best ingredients you can get for anti-aging. Personally, I like to use plant-based stem cell extracts rather than animal stem cells. These active ingredients are like nutrition to your skin and the rejuvenation stimulates cell turnover in your skin, increasing natural collagen production. Serum, unlike other products, focuses on your skin cells rather than just the skin itself. For me, I love serums the most!

CoZi serum works so well because the active ingredients absorb into your skin immediately. It is very rich in amino acid extracts from hibiscus and has apple stem cells and carries many antioxidant properties to fight the free radicals from environmental damage. If you want to address fine lines and wrinkles, it's a product that you will find the most effective. Many of my clients use serum in their regimen and see the results they're looking for! CoZi serum has growth factors that will help to renew and repair the skin. Our serum is my little genie in a bottle!

Serums that have Vitamin A are best for anti-aging and acne. It works to constantly resurface your skin by cell turnover. Vitamin A, also called retinoids, is used in many products for acne clients, but also aging clients. 'Retin-A' is prescribed by a dermatologist which derives from retinoids, but with retinoic acid. It works in the same matter, to resurface the skin, but in a much harsher way due to the chemicals and toxicity. I don't recommend this to my clients for the most part because I see the harsh conditions the skin goes under and can irritate the skin more rather than working for them. I see my clients come back with flaky skin and dryness since the skin can't rejuvenate fast enough. I also recommend my clients to stay away from hydroquinone because it is a harsh whitening agent. Many people use it for lightening pigmentation and age spots. There are great alternatives for natural lightening like Licorice extract and Kojic acid. Vitamin C works best for flat spots like melasma or age spots.


☐    Eye Cream

Eye cream is the most important product for anti-aging. The first sign of aging starts around the eye area (those pesky crow's feet that come in) because the eye area is so delicate. It's the most difficult area to revise the fine lines and wrinkles. So ALWAYS keep this area hydrated because there is not a lot of fat or muscle in this area of our face. The reason I always put eye cream before moisturizer is because you apply with the smallest molecule products first and work your way up. Many people jump to Botox or plastic surgery when they start seeing wrinkles. I am not completely opposed to this, BUT, including something as simple as eye cream in your regimen will slow down, prevent, and aide your skin in a much less invasive and natural way. That's why I always say, use eye cream day and night at whatever age you want in order to prevent aging.

The CoZi eye cream works in multiple areas to prevent aging. It has nanotechnology, which uses smaller molecules to penetrate deeper into the skin. Nanotechnology is amazing! A machine makes the molecules smaller than normal, which can bring nutrition to more layers of skin rather than only the surface. There are Vitamin E and Omegas in the cream to keep the skin hydrated and micronized 23 karat mineral mica to fight off sun damage and reflect UV rays. It all works together to fight and hydrate, but is NOT a greasy product at all. Many of my clients say that this eye cream is the only one where they actually see results. The two products I really think are important to invest in are serum and eye cream. Even if you are a budget shopper or get your products cheaper, it's important to invest a little in these two.


☐    Moisturizer

Moisturizers are like 'the icing on the cake' at the end of your regimen. It's the very last thing that you put on at night- for the morning, put your SPF on top of the moisturizer. For me, moisturizers need to have active ingredients because they protect your skin from environmental damage- free radicals and nurtures your skin when your skin is rejuvenating at night. That is the reason why we use antioxidant ingredients in moisturizers. It usually is the most expensive product, along with serums. There is no 'one moisturizer fits all', it has to be based on your skin-type. For example, I have dry skin, and when I don't use moisturizer, more fine lines show on my face.

I want to break down free radicals, antioxidants, and our skin barrier function here because this is what your moisturizer should target. Free radicals are naturally occurring molecules of your cell function. Many times, they are triggered or sped up from environmental damage like pollution, smoke, diet, alcohol, and chemicals. The bad cells start taking over the good cells and your skin won't reproduce as much as it used to. It becomes a negative reaction. Free radicals need to use antioxidants to help fight against this negative reaction. It's like supplements for your skin through foods like berries, green teas, and more. The antioxidant will soak up those free radicals like a sponge and that is why it's so important for it to be in your moisturizer.

Our skin barrier function is the outermost layer of our epidermis. We have three main layers: epidermis, dermis, and hypodermis. The skin barrier function is like a seal on your skin to fight harsh conditions, like these free radicals I just explained. The dermis is to produce oils, and the hypodermis stores fat and connective tissues. During some seasonal changes, our skin barrier function goes off, and it's completely normal. You can get tightness, dryness, and flaky skin during this transitional period. If you over-exfoliate, use too many products, or do lots of chemical treatments, etc. then you jeopardize its health and functionality.

With my skincare line, our number one seller is the CoZi Blueberry Cream. It has blueberries, green tea, and grape skin which are the highest in antioxidants. Then there is coQ10 for toning. I recommend this product to everyone that is fighting fine lines, dehydration, lack of 'glow' in your skin, and if you have harsh environmental conditions. It's a high impact product with ingredients that I would look for in a moisturizer. Some moisturizers are a 2-in-1, like a day cream with sunscreen in it. When you do a 2-in-1, you compromise the potential of some of the ingredients. Our skin is very complex and we need products to work for our skin, not how you want your skin to work with the products. For example, I have a moisturizer for the face. I have a neck and décolleté cream. They are separate because I want to have different active ingredients to target different reasons.

Moisturizers need a binding agent that keeps the water from evaporating. We DO NOT want mineral oil; it keeps water from evaporating! Most times, this binding agent is too heavy for younger skin.Coconut oil is another oil that I do not recommend using as a moisturizer. Be cautious with it! It seals your body and skin to keep the moisturizer in, but DOES NOT penetrate into nourishing your skin or allowing it to breathe. Oxygen needs to go in and out of our follicles and coconut oil does not allow your follicles to breathe, creating bacteria and irritation stuck in that space. I don't recommend it on your face, but it can still be great for your body and hair is okay.

- SPF

SPF is huge if you want to prevent sun damage and wrinkles! I can't emphasize this enough. SPF is the number one anti-aging product that is inexpensive and works for all ages, starting when you are a baby. If you want to prevent your skin from all kinds of skin disorders, sunscreen is a good start. Make sure you find a good **face** sunscreen for your skin-type. Certain ingredients may be oiler/dryer for your face so be mindful of the one you choose.

With SPF, the higher the number actually doesn't mean the better the protection- higher SPF means the protection extends over a longer period of time. I highly recommend SPF 30 or higher because SPF 30 is the most decent sunscreen you can get with UV coverage. Anything lower cannot protect your skin. If your skin is more reactive to the sun, then it's okay to get a higher SPF. I personally like to use higher SPF on the weekends when I spend more time outside. I will say it again: A common misconception is that you put it on at the beginning of the day and you're good. NO. You HAVE to re-apply throughout the day when you are outside!

*SIDE NOTE:* Be cognisant that SPF sunscreen is not good for the environment or the oceans. When you go to the beach and spray all your SPF sunscreen on, it leaks off into the ocean and damages sea life. When you go to the beach, try to use less sunscreen and more sun protection like umbrellas, hats, sunglasses. You can practice less sun exposure in your day-to-day life as well (:

**At-home facials are total self-care treatment. Stop your busy life schedule to take care of YOU. Spend time for yourself and love yourself. I teach all my clients to do home facials twice a week to maintain their beautiful results from their professional facial. That IS the secret of healthy glowing skin. It IS an essential. Pay attention to your skin, show it love, nurture it, and give it facials!**

☐ Exfoliator

Exfoliating is very important when you are 21+ because as we age, our cell turnover slows down and the turnover rate is not as quick. I always recommend the CoZi Enzyme Peel because that's the most effective and gentle way for people of all ages. It derives from fruit enzymes rather than harsh chemicals to remove everything from your face. It's like a little monster eating and dissolving the dead skin. It's amazing! If you have acne prone skin, it is very important to properly exfoliate so the dead skin doesn't sit on top of your pores and clog up your skin. Many people have milia, the small whiteheads that appear on your skin. This is directly caused by clogged pores and dead skin not being removed. I recommend exfoliating twice a week and follow it up with a mask. You can have a thousand-dollar product, but it doesn't mean it will penetrate and or be as effective as it should be without exfoliating.

☐    Masks

Masks give that little 'extra care' to your regimen when you need it, like a little self spa day! Some people use masks for hydration, anti-aging, or for acne control. Sometimes you just need that little extra exfoliation and hydration that your daily regimen isn't giving you. My routine for masks is twice a week after I use an exfoliator. I do the exfoliator first to remove the dead skin so the mask goes on my fresh new skin. You want to manually remove (gently) the dead skin every so often so that your skin doesn't build it up.

Masks are concentrated ingredients so it's effective, but you can't do it every day depending on what it's for. For example, clay masks are very drying and not good to use every day. Collagen masks are hydrating, and good to use everyday if your skin needs it. I feel you need to be extra cautious of what masks you are using. If it doesn't identify as your skin-type need, it can backfire on you.

If you have oily skin, use a clay mask or ingredients that purify the skin. My skincare line carries an Anti-Blemish clay mask that works great to detox impurities and excess oil. I have clients with papule acne (pesky little bumps) and pustules (common pimples) that absolutely love this product. Antiseptic Sulfur is a key ingredient in my mask, which really helps improve acne skin-types. But remember, if you use a clay mask every single day, it will strip away all your healthy oils. You have to moderate when you use these more concentrated products. If you have dry skin and you want an anti-aging, I recommend my Collagen Mask- and I use it ALL the time. I don't just use it twice. For example, I always bring it with me when I travel and the first thing I do when I check in:  wash my face and put on the collagen mask. The airplane is sooo dehydrating to your skin!

# <u>You Are What You Eat!</u>

When you have problematic skin, whether it be aging, acne, etc. there are more ways to treat it than just products. I want to share knowledge on food alternatives that are healthy, safe, and natural to help you achieve healthier skin. Skin will be more impacted internally than just externally. We are made up of 70% water in our body. It goes without saying that hydration is important. There is no amount of product you can put on your face that will have the same effect as drinking water. One of my favorite sayings, "beauty is inside and out." What you intake in your body is what you put on your skin and you are what you eat. I incorporate nutrition and diet into my practice because it is so important to skincare. The beginning of good skin starts with good health and that can't be emphasized enough. I recommend plant-based diet not only because it's better for your body, but it is also better for the environment.

In my eating-practice, I select a plant-based diet, following a 80/20 rule, 80% vegetables and 20% other. Sometimes I go by 70/30 to increase my protein intake. You really just have to listen to your body and what it is telling you. I recommend "eating the rainbow", meaning the more colors of vegetables that you eat, the more you benefit from the various nutritions. I intentionally set my meal planning weekly based on my lifestyle and skin condition. I struggle with dry skin and have a tendency of aging faster due to my genetics. So I eat a lot of healthy fats like avocado oil, flaxseed oil, and I'm not shy of it. If I don't eat healthy fats for my body, it will just dry out like a prune. I eat a lot of collagen as well because my body lacks the collagen needed to keep my youth. Chicken bone broth has lots of collagen in the bones- I will give the recipe later on. When you're older though, it is better to eat plant-based fats rather than animal fats.

I'm grateful to live in California because they have very fresh seasonal produce. I like to pick on the seasonal fruits and vegetables because it goes with the seasons and nurtures your body in a natural way. We are all living beings, and plants require many of the same things that we do. If a plant thrives in a certain season, I believe it supplies the right nutrients and vitamins that your skin needs to thrive in that season as well. It helps our bodies adjust to the shifting environment. Another tip, when you are grocery shopping, always check the expiration date on your foods. Research the brands that you buy in. Consumerism is a choice and we get to dictate what companies are the best for us. I try to stay away from packaged foods, even if it has simple ingredients because it's better to eat everything fresh. I don't even pre-cut my vegetables because they oxidize quicker which changes the nutrition content in them. But with busy schedules, it is not easy to prepare everything from scratch when you get home from work. The truth is, being healthy is a luxury and it doesn't come easy.

In every consultation, I like to educate my clients on how to get their skin better at home, starting with food. I try to understand their lifestyle and eating habits to help them adjust. For acne clients, the biggest thing to stay away from is sugar, dairy, and gluten. These three food subjects are infamous for causing problems with our bodies. They cause inflammation, redness, and acne. Most cocktails and wine are high in sugars. Not many people know or even incorporate their sugar/caloric intake from the alcohol they drink. One glass of red wine averages 125 calories and .9grams of sugar. A dirty martini is 240 calories and 11.5grams of sugar. 'The 2015 Dietary Guidelines for Americans recommend limiting added sugar intake to no more than 10 percent of daily calories, which is about 12 teaspoons, or 50 grams.' For me, that's even a lot and I try to do less in my diet. It not only brings toxins into your body, making your liver work harder, but inflames your skin. I've seen skin transform after a 30 day detox with less acne, dark circles, and overall dullness disappears.

I started drinking warm lemon water in the morning to alkalize your body and a daily detox boost. You have to train your intestines before you take on the whole lemon and work your way up. Start with half a lemon with 16oz of warm water, and then by the end of the month, begin using the whole lemon with your 16oz of warm water. Also, I always recommend a probiotic because they boost your gut flora and improve gut health, especially for women. Probiotics are a good bacteria that helps eliminate the bad bacteria in your gut, keeping everything in balance and helping bowel movement. A lot of skin issues come from gut health and the digestive system. In Chinese medicine, we always say that everything is connected. When you are having an issue with an internal part of your body, it will reflect on the external. You can get probiotics from many different foods rather than just taking it in a pill form. Unsweetened yogurt, sauerkraut, kimchi, kombucha, and basically anything that is fermented food has all natural probiotics.

For dry skin, I always recommend eating more healthy fats like avocado, flaxseed oil, salmon, etc. and make sure you drink a lot of water. Don't be shy of eating fats, but be cognisant of what is a healthy fat and unhealthy fat. A lot of my clients complain about dry skin and use heavy moisturizer. This heavy moisturizer does not work! The molecules are usually too large to penetrate the skin deep enough to solve the root of the problem. I look at eating healthy fats like putting oils from underneath the skin and working its way out.  It's more important to stay away from the sun if you have dry skin and take daily supplements that include Vitamin D and fish oil.

If you suffer from Eczema, then you know that it acts up when the weather starts to cool down. Our bodies start to dry with the colder temperatures and cause a flare up. Even if you don't have Eczema, you'll notice this dryness in your skin. There are foods that you can eat to help with this. Pumpkins are great to eat baked, steamed, and boiled (and they're also in season!) Fruits like pears, apples, cranberries, and grapefruit are good too. If you want to stay away from too much sugar, find foods with omega-3 fatty acids. Fish and seafood are rich with omega-3's! Or leafy greens, red onions, peppers, broccoli, and green tea. These will all help you naturally help and prevent flare-ups of eczema and help with the dryness you're experiencing in the weather change.

One thing I want everyone to take home is to **cook your own collagen bone broth**. Collagen is the best natural source to maintain youthfulness and prevent aging. When you produce more collagen in your body by ingesting it, it stimulates it to grow on its own. I don't particularly trust collagen pills or powder because you never really know where they are getting it from. I always use an organic chicken, and when I can I purchase from local farmers, not mass production. The bones, ligaments, and skin of a chicken have so much collagen in it. In fact, chicken collagen is used to heal arthritis because it fights inflammation and pain. I use the whole chicken when I make a bone broth soup because every part of the chicken is beneficial to your skin. The hardest part of this recipe is removing the fat in between the skin and the muscle. The best way to do this is to leave the chicken broth in the fridge overnight and the next day remove the top layer that is hardened fat. If you're not a fan of the skin, it's okay to take it out.

I have two ways of making this soup: my normal, and my Chinese herb. In the normal chicken soup, I put lots of ginger and garlic with the whole chicken in a big pot! I cook it for two hours in a pressure cooker, then put it in the refrigerator overnight. The next day, I remove the top layer of fat that formed on the top. I put it back on the stove and when it is boiling, I add in shitake mushrooms and a little bit of salt. Sometimes I remove some of the broth with the mushrooms and add kale to make a kale soup with my collagen broth. If you can't finish your soup in a reasonable time (eating a whole chicken for one person takes a while) you can easily put it in a container and freeze it until you're ready for more. There are so many variations on how to make a big pot of bone broth soup!

☐     Botanicals

Botanicals are a plant-based additive we include in all kinds of products, including skincare products. This substance comes from all the fruits, vegetables, herbs, roots, flowers, etc. that we ingest every day. I love botanicals. I believe that our bodies are able to live solely off the Earth if we eat and take care of it properly. I have used and studied many Chinese herbs that we use in our medicine and seen their capability in healing. The Earth provides us with natural healing remedies, and we just need to use them correctly. You do need technology to make the components on how to absorb it into our skin topically, so it is now a mixture of natural and human innovation.

Every ingredient that I list in my products that comes from the Earth will work from the natural source just as good. When I use Apple Stem cells in my anti-aging serum, it's because the apple itself is good for anti-aging. For sensitive skin, I love using chamomile as an ingredient in skincare products because it is soothing and calming. My theory is that if we extract it for our topical products, why not focus on ingesting it too? I focus highly on botanicals in my practice and my products. I use all natural ingredient extracts in my products, and don't add parabens because I really truly believe that the Earth provides everything we need to care for ourselves.

I don't believe in traumatizing the skin to renew. Eventually, it won't have much structure to rebuild from if you're too invasive. When you nurture yourself from the blood cells, from the root, then we can create a strong skin structure. Each botanical will serve a different purpose. Some are for treating skin conditions, some are good for anti-aging, some relieve inflammation, and you really need a deeper understanding of how it will serve your skin-type. Look for these botanicals not only in your products, but more so in your diet!

Here's a start to understanding botanicals and their purpose for your skin:

- *Leaves & Flowers*
    - Chamomile - good for soothing and calming the skin. Reduces redness and diminishes acne breakouts.
    - Calendula - comes from the pot marigold flower. It has antiseptic properties which work great for

preventing acne, stimulating collagen growth, and helping with dry skin.
- Red and white teas - good for UV protection at the root of your skin.
- Clove leaf - emulsifies oil and debris throughout the day without stripping the healthy oil. It's ideal for reducing blackheads, pustules, and pimples from oily skin.
- Aloe Vera - anti inflammatory

- *Oils*
  - Avocado oil - healthy fats that help with dry skin and acne skin.
  - Sunflower oil - a non-comedogenic oil, highly absorbent, great moisturizer, and great for all skin-types because it is non-irritating and doesn't clog pores.
  - Rosehip seed oil - carries provitamin A (beta-carotene) and carries the essential fatty acids (omega-6 and omega-3). It is pressed from the fruit and seeds of the rose plant. It helps with anti-aging due to the vitamin A that helps cell turnover.
  - Calendula oil - promotes antifungal, anti inflammatory, and antibacterial. Very useful for healing skin wounds, rashes, and soothing eczema.
  - Sea buckthorn Extract - helps your skin heal from wounds and sunburns. It promotes elasticity and fights dryness. Works well if you have sensitive or irritated skin.

- *Fruits*
  - Blueberries - high in antioxidants, aid anti-aging by reducing fine lines, and provide moisture for dry or mature skin.
  - Oranges - Great for moisture retention

- *Vegetables:*

- ○ Pumpkins seeds - gives hydration and soothes inflamed skin.
  - ○ Cucumbers - Great for detoxing the skin and provides healing properties.

- *Roots:*
  - ○ Ginger - anti inflammatory
  - ○ Ginseng - reactivates your skin epidermal cells
  - ○ Turmeric - anti inflammatory

# <u>Care For Yourself. Inside and Outside of the Spa</u>

*"Self love, self care, self authority, and self acceptance. Go as far as you can and run with it."*

Many people ask me what the one best thing they can do to take care of their skin and I always say there is no one best thing. It is a combination of your daily habits, products, and diet. They all play equal roles in your skincare, and your health! Because skincare is not just beauty, it is your HEALTH. And each skin-type needs to be treated properly if you ever want to see results using all three ways.

Now that we've gone through the different kinds of products, how to create your regimen, and beneficial foods to eat, I lastly want to stress self care. I have focused my practice highly around self-care. This entails mental and physical health. Living a balanced life is key! I call Sunday's #SelfcareSunday because it's a great day to focus on yourself. This doesn't mean putting more time aside for your family or significant other (even though they are very important too), but solely for yourself. Even just one hour. Maybe you have a hobby, or you like to cook, meditate, yoga, take a long bubble bath, go for a run, watch the sunset, do a face mask, watch that movie you've put off, read a book. THAT is self-care. Setting aside a moment for yourself out of your busy schedule to just be at peace.

Some people, like myself, struggle with this because you feel guilty or wrong for focusing on yourself. But when you aren't taking care of yourself, you cannot give your best to the people around you. Happiness starts from yourself and shines outward. When you gravitate energy towards the things that bring you happiness, you're able to share that joy with the people around you. Everyone needs a little pampering. Everyone needs to keep good hygiene and keep their appearance healthy. A little exfoliation and hydration. People always say they don't have enough time in the day to self-care. In reality, it only takes 10-15 minutes to do something for yourself.

Everyone has 10-15 minutes to give to themselves. Those 10-15 minutes are crucial to your skincare and mental health!

On a last note, I want this book to remove the lense of the skincare industry and all their marketing techniques. I want everyone reading to stop filling up that drawer with products you rarely use. Always buying, buying, buying with no improvement. This book is for all the people coming into my workplace being traumatized with the skincare information they've been told. You've either let your guard down completely or built such a high wall you don't know what to believe. So this book is about your own judgement. Self educate and make your own choice for your skin and for yourself. Always know there is a place to reach out if you need help!

I don't only want this book to be about skincare, I want this to be about a journey. Starting at 17, I made this into my life. Now, a part of my skincare knowledge is for everyone to know. And this is you giving yourself permission to educate yourself. It is about dedicating your money, time, and love to yourself. You don't have to have perfect skin without any blemishes or disorders to be beautiful. Learn to love yourself inside and out and that will radiate on your skin. Skincare led me to my purpose, a healer and esthetician. It gave me a purpose to be a woman, to be independent. I believe in just showing up and trying in the most loving and positive way possible. It has always created this space for me to be soft and caring. I'm so grateful for my clients and for my job.

Thank you for letting me share with you.

CoCo Pai